NOURISH

&

THRIVE

20 MENOPAUSE
DIET RECIPES
FOR A
HEALTHY TRANSITION

DR JOYCE A. MOORE

1

This book does not offer psychiatric or medical advice; it is just intended for informational and educational purposes. If you have specific concerns about your medical or mental health, please speak with a trained expert.

Copyright © 2024 by Dr Joyce A. Moore

amazon.com/author/joyceamoore

All rights reserved.

Gratitude

Writing *Nourish and Thrive* has been a deeply fulfilling journey, and I am immensely grateful to everyone who contributed to making this book a reality.

To my readers—thank you for trusting me as a guide on your wellness journey. Your commitment to embracing a healthier lifestyle during this transformative stage of life is truly inspiring.

To my family—your unwavering support, encouragement, and belief in my vision have been a source of strength and motivation. I am beyond grateful for your love and patience.

To the health and nutrition experts who have shared valuable insights and research—your work continues to inspire and educate, helping countless individuals navigate menopause with confidence and ease.

Finally, to every woman embracing this phase of life with grace and resilience—you are the

reason this book exists. May these recipes
nourish your body, uplift your spirit, and
empower you to thrive.

With heartfelt gratitude,

JOYCE A. MOORE

Content

14. Almond Butter and Banana Smoothie
Bowl
15. Eggplant and Chickpea Curry
16. Chia Seed Pudding with Berries
17. Baked Cod with Lemon-Herb Crust
18. Greek Yogurt Parfait with Nuts and Berries
19. Lentil and Vegetable Soup
20. Roasted Brussels Sprouts with Balsamic
Glaze
Conclusion

Introduction

Welcome to this culinary journey designed to guide and empower women through the transformative phase of menopause.

This book is more than just a collection of recipes; it's a comprehensive guide crafted with care to support your well-being during this significant life transition.

As you navigate the complexities of menopause, "Nourish & Thrive" stands as your companion, offering not only delicious and nourishing recipes but also insights into how mindful nutrition can contribute to a healthier, more vibrant you.

Embracing Change with Wholesome Nutrition

Menopause is a natural and inevitable phase in a woman's life, and the dietary choices we make during this time can play a crucial role in managing the symptoms and promoting overall health.

"Nourish & Thrive" was created with the concept that embracing change should be an exciting and stimulating experience. Through a carefully chosen collection of recipes, we hope to demonstrate that nourishing your body can be a pleasurable and transforming aspect of your menopausal journey.

The Culinary Pattern of "Nourish & Thrive"

This book weaves together a culinary that celebrates wholesome, nutrient-dense ingredients.

From flavorful salads to comforting soups, energizing smoothies to satisfying main courses, each recipe is thoughtfully designed to address the nutritional needs specific to menopause.

Drawing inspiration from diverse cuisines, "Nourish & Thrive" offers a variety of options to suit different tastes and preferences, ensuring that every meal is a moment of nourishment and joy.

9

"Nourish & Thrive" goes beyond the plate, providing insights into how dietary choices can positively impact hormonal balance, manage symptoms, and contribute to overall well-being. Embrace this opportunity to nourish your body and thrive during menopause. Let each recipe in this collection be a step towards a healthier, more vibrant you.

As we embark on this culinary and wellness journey together, may "Nourish & Thrive" be your trusted guide to a wholesome and joy-filled transition through menopause. Here's to embracing change, nourishing your body, and thriving during this transformative phase of life.

Navigating Menopause with Empathy and Expertise

Menopause is a chapter filled with special challenges and experiences, and this book is written with an understanding of the journey's complexities. The recipes on these pages are not only intended to excite your taste senses, but also to address typical menopausal problems such as hormone imbalances, sleep disorders, and changes in metabolism.

A Symphony of Flavors and Wellness

Each recipe is a harmonious blend of flavors and wellness. From vibrant spices that enliven the senses to nutrient-rich ingredients that support overall health, every dish is a symphony of tastes and benefits.

Discover the joy of crafting meals that not only satiate your palate but also contribute to your overall well-being, helping you navigate the challenges of menopause with grace and vitality.

Through Culinary Exploration

Consider this book not just a cookbook, but a culinary companion on your journey toward empowerment and well-being. Explore the art of meal preparation as a form of self-care, where each ingredient is chosen with intention and every recipe becomes an opportunity to nourish both body and spirit. It encourages you to embrace the kitchen as a space for self-discovery and empowerment during this transformative phase of life.

Beyond the Kitchen: A Holistic Approach

In addition to amazing dishes, "Nourish & Thrive" takes a comprehensive approach to menopause, including advice on lifestyle choices, mindfulness techniques, and nutritional insights. This book wants to be your comprehensive resource, providing you with the tools and information to help you make educated decisions that will benefit your menopausal transition. Let "Nourish & Thrive" take you through this gastronomic and health trip. This resource not only enhances the flavor of your food, but it also enriches your menopausal journey with vigor, balance, and a celebration of the robust woman you are becoming.

20 Delicious Menopause Diet Recipes

1. Hormone-Balancing Smoothie:

Ingredients:

1 cup mixed berries (blue berries, strawberries, and raspberries)

1/2 cup Greek yogurt (unsweetened)

1 cup almond milk (unsweetened)

1 teaspoon honey (optional, for sweetness)

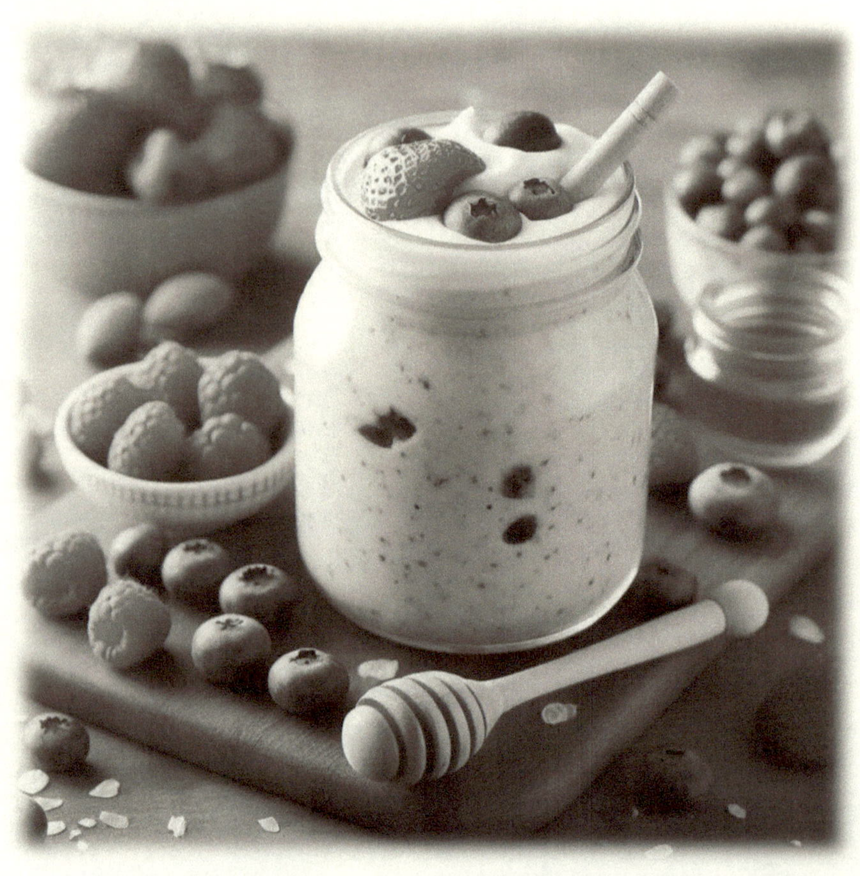

Place the mixed berries in a blender.

16

Add ground flaxseeds, Greek yogurt, and almond milk to the blender.

If desired, drizzle in honey for sweetness.

Blend all the ingredients until smooth and well combined.

Pour the smoothie into a glass and drink immediately.

Benefits to the Menopausal Woman:

1. Antioxidant Powerhouse:

Berries: Packed with antioxidants, berries combat oxidative stress linked to hormonal changes during menopause. Antioxidants help neutralize free radicals, supporting overall health.

2. Omega-3 Fatty Acid Boost:

Flaxseeds are rich in alpha-linolenic acid (ALA), a plant-based omega-3 fatty acid. Omega-3s contribute to hormonal balance and are associated with reduced inflammation, easing menopausal symptoms.

3. Probiotics for Gut Health:

Greek Yogurt: Greek yogurt contains probiotics, which maintain a healthy gut microbiota. Maintaining gut health is essential during menopause because it affects hormone metabolism and nutrition absorption.

4. Nutrient-rich almond milk:

Almond milk contains vitamin E, magnesium, and calcium. These nutrients play roles in bone health, mood regulation, and overall well-being during menopause.

5. Optional sweetness without refined sugars:

Honey: If chosen, honey adds natural sweetness without refined sugars. This can be beneficial for women looking to manage their sugar intake during menopause.

How It Supports Hormonal Balance:

This hormone-balancing smoothie is a tailored blend of ingredients designed to address specific needs during menopause. Antioxidant-rich berries combat oxidative stress, while omega-3 fatty acids from flaxseeds contribute to hormonal equilibrium. The inclusion of probiotic-rich Greek yogurt supports gut health, influencing hormonal metabolism. Almond milk provides essential nutrients, and the optional honey allows for sweetness without compromising nutritional goals.

Incorporate this smoothie into your routine to enjoy a delicious and nutrient-packed way to support hormonal balance during the menopausal transition

2. Kale and Quinoa Power Salad

Ingredients:

2 cups kale, finely chopped

1 cup of cooked Quinoa, cooled

1/2 cup cherry tomatoes, halved

1/4 cup red onion, finely chopped

1 cucumber diced

1/4 cup red onion, finely chopped

1/4 cup feta cheese, crumbled

1/4 cup extra-virgin olive oil

2 tablespoons balsamic vinegar

1 teaspoon Dijon mustard

Salt and pepper to taste

1/4 cup almonds, sliced (optional, for added crunch)

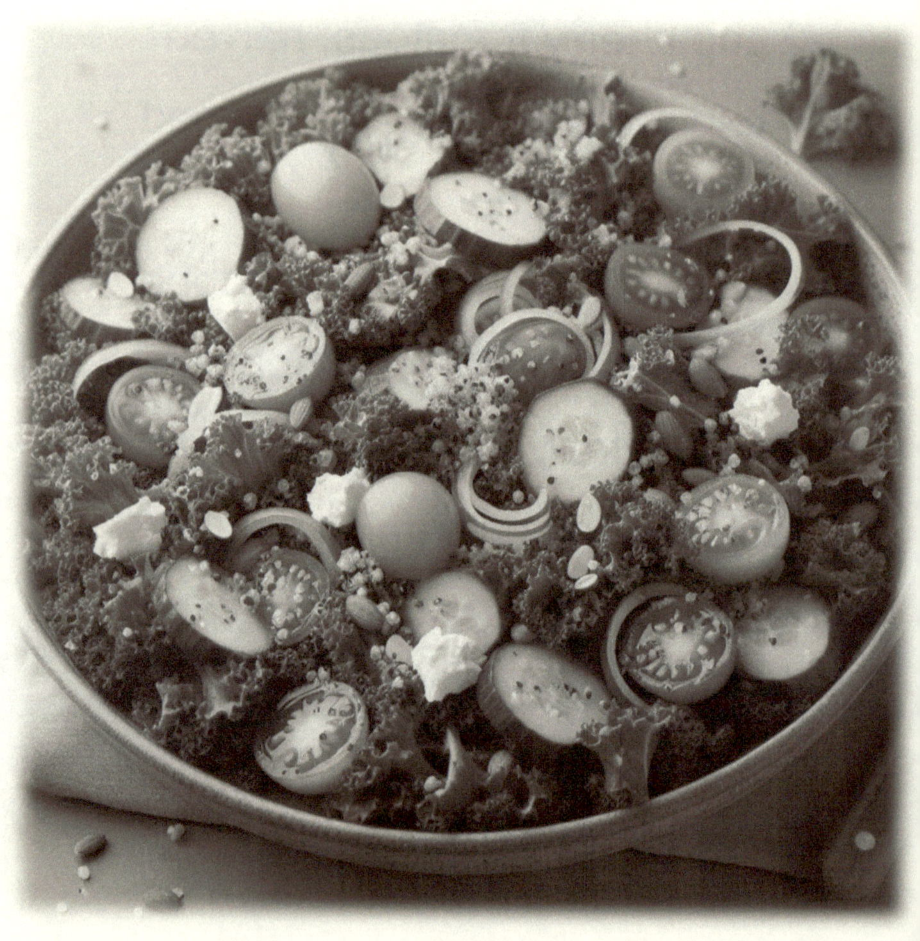

In a large bowl, combine the chopped kale and cooked quinoa.

Add cherry tomatoes, cucumber, red onions, and crumbled feta cheese into the bowl.

In a small bowl, whisk together olive oil, balsamic vinegar, Dijon mustard, salt, and pepper to create the dressing.

Pour the dressing over the salad and toss until all ingredients are well coated.

Allow the salad to rest for a few minutes so that the flavors can mix together. If desired, sprinkle sliced almonds on top for added crunch just before serving.

This nutrient-rich, delicious Kale and Quinoa power salad is best served cold.

Benefits to the Menopausal Woman:

1. High in Fiber: Kale and quinoa are rich in dietary fiber, promoting digestive health and helping manage weight during menopause.
2. Nutrient-Dense: The combination of kale, quinoa, and vegetables provides a wide array of vitamins and minerals essential for overall well-being.
3. Healthy Fats: Olive oil and feta cheese contribute heart-healthy monounsaturated fats,

supporting cardiovascular health.

4. Protein Powerhouse: Quinoa is a complete protein source, and feta cheese adds protein to support muscle health.
5. Antioxidant-Rich: Cherry tomatoes and kale offer antioxidants, helping combat oxidative stress associated with hormonal changes.
6. Bone Health: Kale contains calcium, vital for bone health, which becomes especially important during menopause.
7. Balanced Flavors: The balsamic-Dijon dressing provides a perfect balance of tanginess and depth, enhancing the overall enjoyment of the salad.

This Kale and Quinoa Power Salad is not only a delightful culinary experience but also a nutritional powerhouse designed to nourish and support women during the menopausal transition.

3. Spiced Sweet Potato Soup:

Ingredients:

2 large sweet potatoes, peeled and diced

1 carrot, peeled and chopped

1 onion, diced

2 cloves garlic, minced

1 teaspoon ground turmeric

1 teaspoon ground ginger

½ teaspoon cinnamon

4 cups vegetable broth

1 tablespoon olive oil

Salt and pepper to taste

Coconut milk (optional, for garnish)

Fresh cilantro (optional, for garnish)

Preparation:

In a large cooking saucepan, heat the olive oil over medium heat.

Add the chopped onion and heat until softened.

Add minced garlic, ground turmeric, ground ginger, and cinnamon to the pot. Stir and heat for 1-2 minutes,

27

until aromatic.

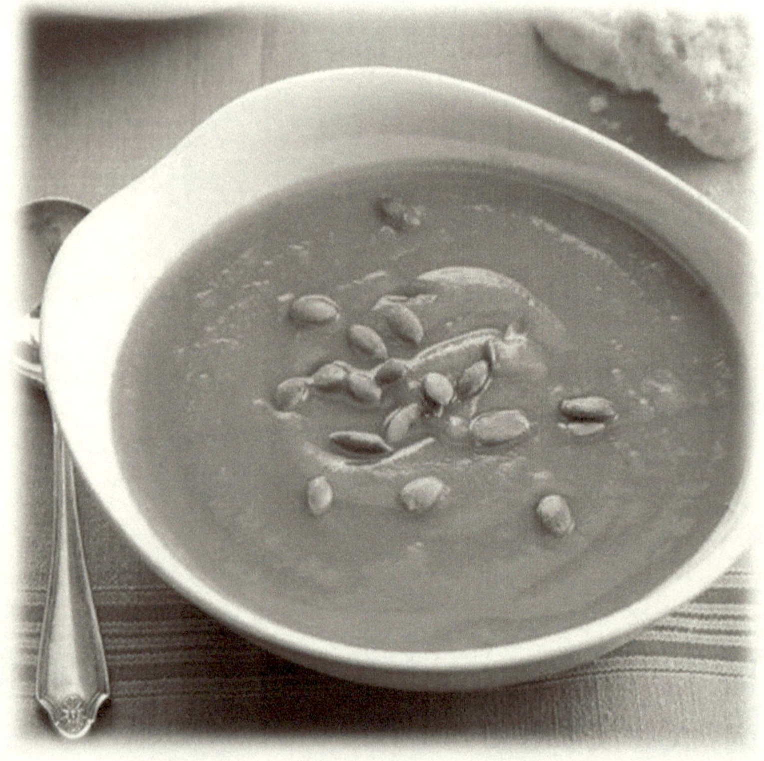

Add diced sweet potatoes and carrots to the pot.

Season well, with salt and pepper. Stir to evenly coat the veggies with the seasonings.

Pour in the veggie broth and boil.

28

Reduce the heat to low, cover, and cook for approximately 20–25 minutes, or until the sweet potatoes are cooked.

Use an immersion blender to puree the soup until smooth. Alternatively, transfer the soup in batches to a blender and blend until smooth.

Adjust the seasoning as required. If the soup is too thick, add additional vegetable broth until you get the required consistency.

Serve the soup hot, topped with a swirl of coconut milk and fresh cilantro if preferred.

Benefits for Menopausal Women:

1. Anti-Inflammatory Properties: Turmeric and ginger in the

soup are known for their anti-inflammatory properties, potentially helping to manage inflammation associated with menopausal symptoms.

2. Rich in Vitamin A: Sweet potatoes are rich in beta-carotene, a precursor to vitamin A, which is crucial for immune function, skin health, and vision.

3. Digestive Health: Carrots in the soup contribute to fiber, aiding in digestion and supporting a healthy gut – an important consideration during menopause.

4. Warm and Comforting: The warm temperature and comforting nature of the soup may provide a soothing effect, especially during times of hormonal fluctuations.

5. Blood Sugar Regulation: Cinnamon in the soup may assist in regulating blood sugar levels, potentially beneficial for women experiencing changes in insulin sensitivity during menopause.

6. Hydration: The broth base of the soup helps with hydration, which is essential for overall health and may be particularly relevant during menopause.

7. Heart-Healthy Fats: The optional addition of coconut milk provides healthy fats, supporting cardiovascular health.

This spiced sweet potato soup not only offers a burst of flavors but also brings together ingredients with potential benefits tailored to support women during the menopausal transition.

4. Salmon with Lemon-Dill Sauce:

Ingredients:

4 salmon fillets

2 tablespoons fresh dill, chopped

2 tablespoons lemon juice

1 tablespoon olive oil

2 cloves garlic, minced

Salt and pepper to taste

Lemon wedges for garnish

Preparation:

Preheat the oven to 400°F (200°C). Line a baking sheet with parchment paper.

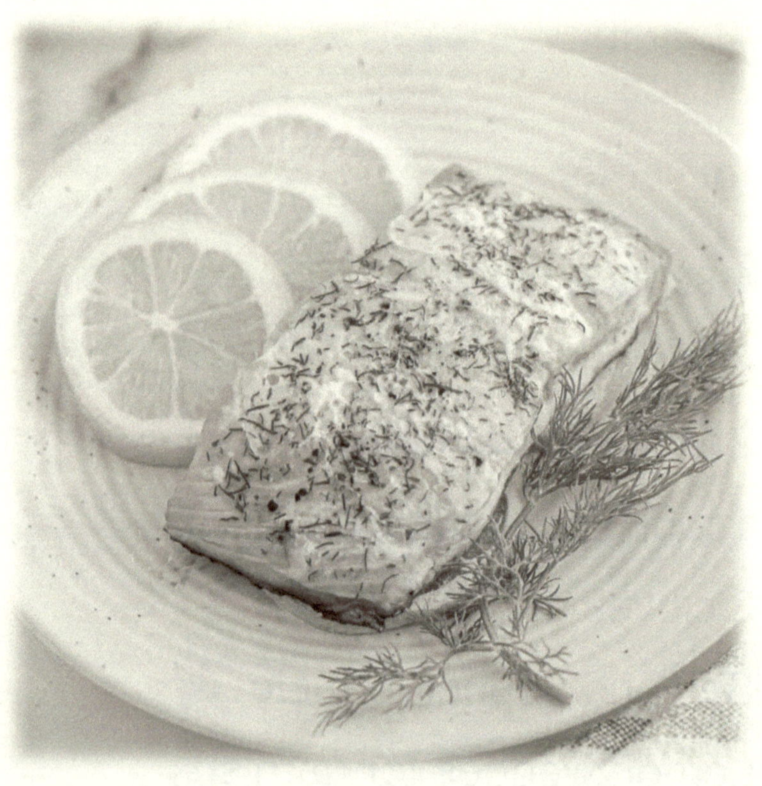

Place salmon fillets on the prepared baking sheet. Season well, with salt and pepper.

In a small bowl, mix chopped dill, lemon juice, olive oil, and minced garlic to create the sauce.

Brush the lemon-dill sauce over each salmon fillet, ensuring an even coating.

Bake in the preheated oven for about 12-15 minutes or until the salmon is cooked through and easily flakes with a fork.

Remove from the oven and garnish with additional fresh dill and lemon wedges.

Serve the salmon hot with your favorite side dishes.

Benefits to Menopausal Women:

1. Omega-3 Fatty Acids: Salmon is rich in omega-3 fatty acids, such as EPA and DHA, which have anti-inflammatory properties and may assist in

managing symptoms associated with hormonal fluctuations during menopause.

2. Heart Health: Omega-3s contribute to cardiovascular health, helping manage cholesterol levels and supporting overall heart function – important considerations during menopause.

3. Protein Power: Salmon is an excellent source of high-quality protein, aiding in muscle maintenance and overall body strength, which becomes increasingly important during and after menopause.

4. Vitamin D Boost: Salmon is a natural source of vitamin D, crucial for calcium absorption and bone health, especially relevant during menopause when bone density may decline.

5. Mood Regulation: Omega-3 fatty acids are associated with mood regulation, potentially providing emotional well-being during times of hormonal changes.

6. Anti-Inflammatory Benefits: The combination of salmon, dill, and garlic provides anti-

inflammatory benefits, potentially assisting in managing inflammation associated with menopausal symptoms.

7. Delicious and Versatile: Salmon with Lemon-Dill Sauce offers a delicious and versatile option that can be easily paired with a variety of nutrient-rich side dishes to create a balanced and satisfying meal.

Incorporating this Salmon with Lemon-Dill Sauce into a menopausal woman's diet provides a delectable and nutritious option that aligns with specific health considerations during this phase of life.

5. Cauliflower and Broccoli Stir-Fry:

Ingredients:

1 small cauliflower, cut into florets

1 broccoli crown, cut into florets

tofu, cubed

2 tablespoons soy sauce (low-sodium)

1 tablespoon sesame oil

2 tablespoons olive oil

3 cloves garlic, minced

1 tablespoon fresh ginger, grated

1 red bell pepper, thinly sliced

1 carrot, julienned

2 green onions, chopped

Sesame oil

brown rice or quinoa, cooked (optional, for serving)

Preparation:

In a large wok or skillet, heat olive oil over medium-high heat. Add the cubed tofu and stir-fry until golden brown. Take away the tofu from the wok and put it aside.

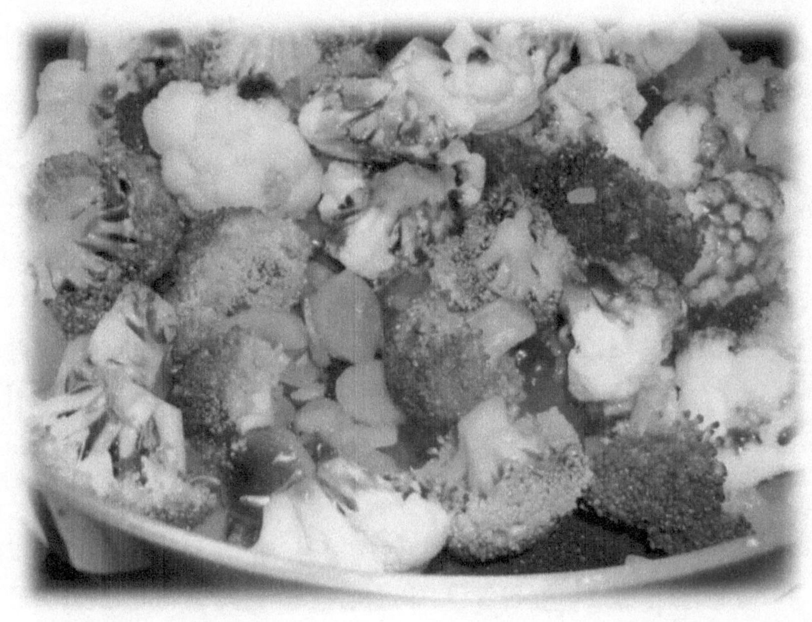

In the same pan, mix sesame oil and minced garlic.

 Sauté for about 1-2 minutes, until fragrant.

Add the cauliflower and broccoli florets to the pan.

Stir-fry the veggies for 3-4 minutes, until they are slightly soft but still crisp.

Add the grated ginger, red bell pepper, and julienned carrot to the pan. Stir-fry for another 2-3 minutes.

Return the cooked tofu to the wok. Pour the soy sauce over the ingredients and stir until well covered and cooked.

Remove from heat and serve with chopped green onions and sesame seeds, if preferred.

Serve the cauliflower and broccoli stir-fry over cooked brown rice or quinoa, if preferred.

Benefits for Menopausal Women:

1. Plant-Based Protein: Tofu in the stir-fry provides plant-

based protein, essential for muscle health and overall well-being, especially during menopause.

2. Cruciferous Vegetables: Cauliflower and broccoli are cruciferous vegetables rich in compounds that may support estrogen balance, an important consideration during menopause.

3. Low-Calorie Option: Cauliflower and broccoli are low in calories and high in fiber, aiding in weight management, which can be a concern during menopause.

4. Vitamin C Boost: Red bell pepper is a rich source of vitamin C, promoting immune health and collagen production for skin support.

5. Healthy Fats: Sesame oil adds a touch of healthy fats, contributing to satiety and supporting heart health.

6. Nutrient Diversity: The diverse array of vegetables in the stir-fry ensures a mix of vitamins, minerals, and antioxidants crucial for overall health during menopause.

7. Quick and Versatile: This stir-fry is a quick and versatile option, allowing for easy customization and adaptation to individual preferences and dietary needs.

Incorporating this cauliflower and broccoli stir-fry into a menopausal woman's diet provides a delicious, nutrient-packed option that aligns with specific health considerations during this transformative phase of life.

6. Avocado and Chickpea Salad:

Ingredients:

2 ripe avocados, diced

1 can (15 oz) chickpeas, washed and drained

1 cup cherry tomatoes, halved

1 cucumber, diced

1/4 cup red onion, finely chopped

1/4 cup feta cheese

 fresh cilantro or parsley.

2 tablespoons extra-virgin olive oil

 balsamic vinegar

Salt and pepper to taste

Optional: Lemon juice for added freshness

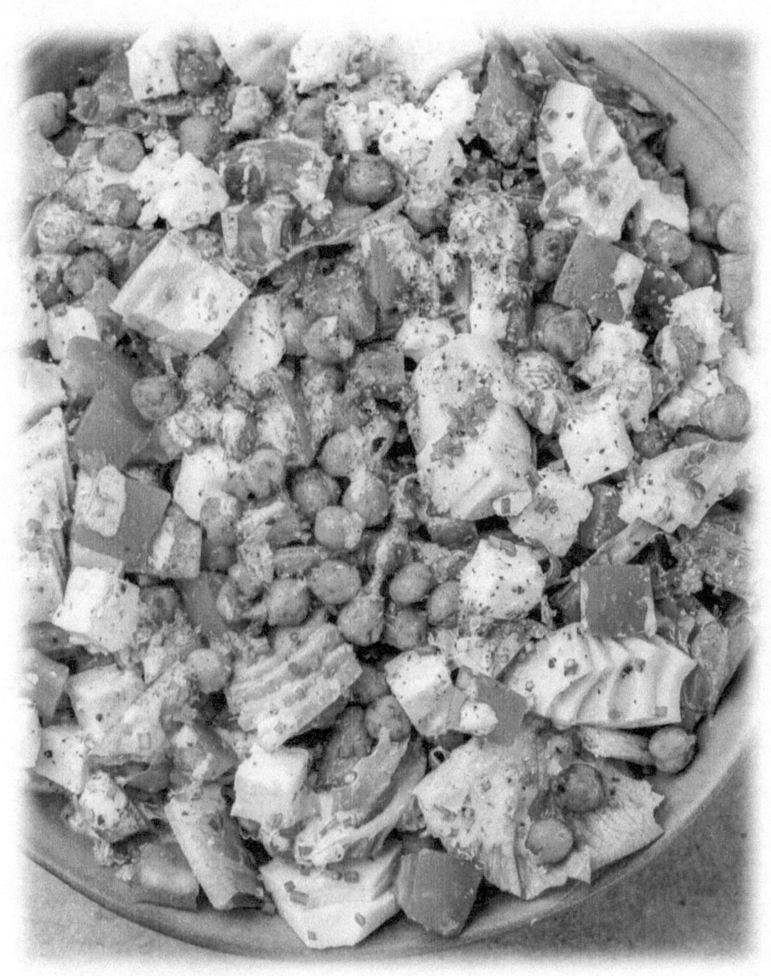

Preparation:

In a large mixing bowl, combine diced avocados, chickpeas, cherry

47

tomatoes, cucumber, red onion, feta cheese, and fresh cilantro or parsley.

In a small bowl, whisk together extra-virgin olive oil, balsamic vinegar, salt, and pepper to create the dressing.

Pour the dressing over the salad items and gently toss until evenly covered.

Refrigerate the salad for 30 minutes before serving to allow flavors to mingle.

Before serving, adjust the salt and pepper to your liking. Serve the avocado and chickpea salad as a refreshing side or a light main dish.

Benefits for Menopausal Women:

1. Avocados include monounsaturated fats, which promote heart health and provide a satisfying touch to salads.
2. Plant-Based Protein: Chickpeas are an excellent source of plant-based protein, crucial for muscle health and overall well-being during menopause.

3. Fiber for Digestive Health: The combination of avocados and chickpeas provides dietary fiber, supporting digestive health and helping manage weight.
4. Hydration Support: Cucumbers in the salad have high water content, aiding in hydration –

an essential consideration during menopause.

5. Rich in antioxidants: cherry tomatoes and fresh herbs contribute antioxidants, combating oxidative stress associated with hormonal changes.
6. Bone Health: Feta cheese adds a touch of calcium, supporting bone health during a phase when maintaining bone density is important.

7. Balanced Nutrition: The diverse mix of nutrients, including vitamins, minerals, and healthy fats, provides balanced nutrition for overall well-being.

8. Low-Glycemic Option: The salad has a low glycemic index, helping regulate blood sugar levels, which can be relevant during menopause.

The Avocado and Chickpea Salad offers a delicious and nutrient-packed option that aligns with specific health considerations for women navigating the menopausal transition.

7. Quinoa-stuffed Bell Peppers:

Ingredients:

4 large bell peppers, cut into halves and seeds removed

1 cup quinoa, rinse

2 cups vegetable broth

1 can (15 oz) black beans, rinse and drain

1 cup corn kernels (fresh or frozen)

1 cup cherry tomatoes, diced

1/2 red onion, finely chopped

2 cloves

2 Garlic minced

1 teaspoon chili powder

Ground cumin

1/2 teaspoon paprika

Salt and pepper to taste

1 cup shredded cheese (cheddar, pepper jack, or your choice)

Fresh cilantro for garnish (optional)

Preparation:

Preheat the oven to 375°F (190°C).

In a medium saucepan, combine the quinoa and vegetable broth.

Bring to a boil, then reduce heat to low, cover, and simmer for 15-20 and liquid is absorbed minutes or until quinoa is cooked

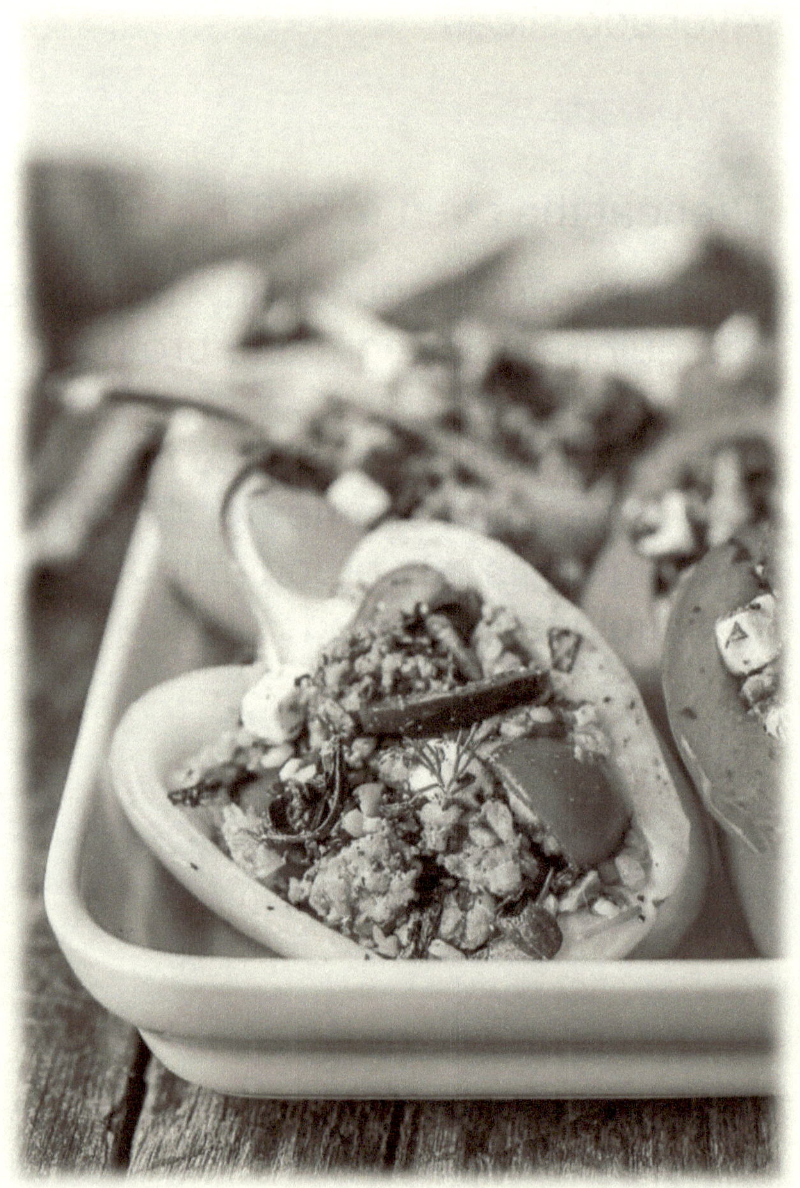

.In a large mixing bowl, combine cooked quinoa, black beans, corn, cherry tomatoes, red onion, minced garlic, ground cumin, chili powder, paprika, salt, and pepper. Mix well.

Put the bell pepper halves on a baking tray. Fill each pepper half with the quinoa mixture.

Top each filled pepper with grated cheese.

Cover the baking dish with foil and bake for 25–30 minutes, or until the peppers are cooked.

If desired, broil for an additional 2-3 minutes to melt and lightly brown the cheese.

Remove from the oven, top with fresh cilantro, and serve with avocado slices if preferred.

1. Plant-Based Protein: Quinoa, black beans, and cheese provide plant-based protein, crucial for muscle health and overall well-being during menopause.

2. Fiber-Rich: Quinoa, black beans, and vegetables contribute to the fiber content, supporting digestive health and weight management.

3. Bone Health: Bell peppers, quinoa, and cheese provide calcium, essential for maintaining bone health during menopause.

4. Anti-Inflammatory Spices: The inclusion of cumin, chili powder, and paprika adds not only flavor but also anti-inflammatory benefits, potentially assisting in managing inflammation associated with menopausal symptoms.

5. Vitamins and Minerals: The diverse mix of vegetables offers a range of vitamins and minerals, contributing to overall nutritional balance.

6. Low-Glycemic Option: Quinoa is a low-glycemic grain, helping regulate blood sugar levels,

which can be beneficial during menopause.

7. Versatile and Customizable: This dish is versatile, allowing for customization based on personal preferences and dietary needs.

Quinoa-Stuffed Bell Peppers offers a wholesome and flavorful option that aligns with the nutritional needs and considerations of women navigating the menopausal transition.

8. Mediterranean Zucchini Boats:

Ingredients:

4 large Courgettes or Zucchini

1 pound lean ground turkey or chicken

1 cup cherry tomatoes, halved

1/2 cup of Kalamata olives, pitted and chopped

1/2 cup crumbled feta cheese

1/4 cup red onion, finely chopped

2 cloves garlic, minced

1 teaspoon dried oregano

Salt and pepper to taste2 tablespoons olive oil

Fresh parsley for garnish (optional)

Lemon wedges for serving (optional)

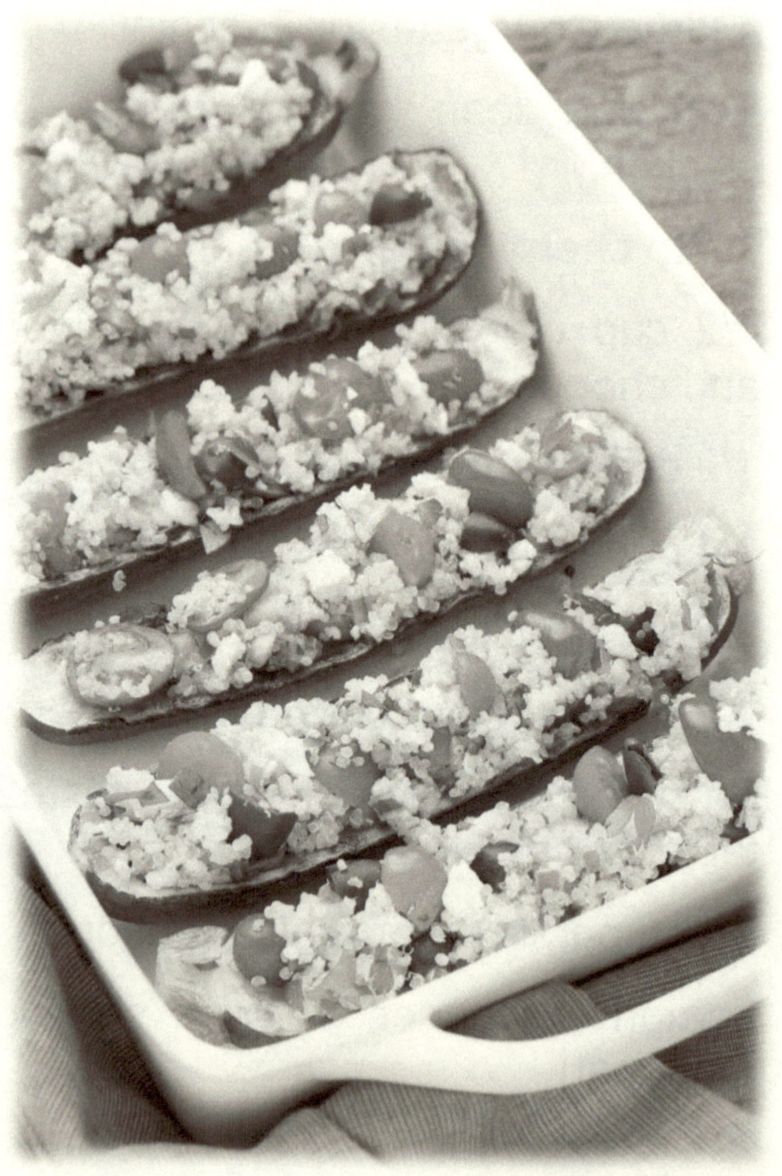

Preparation:

Preheat the oven to 375°F (190°C).

Scoop out the flesh from the zucchini halves, leaving about 1/4-inch-thick shells. Chop the zucchini flesh and set aside.

In a large skillet, heat olive oil over medium heat. Add minced garlic and chopped red onion, sautéing until softened.

Add ground turkey or chicken to the skillet and cook until browned.

Stir in the chopped zucchini flesh, cherry tomatoes, olives, dried oregano, dried basil, salt, and pepper. Cook for an additional 5-7 minutes until the vegetables are delicate.

61

Remove the pan from the heat and mix in the crumbled feta cheese.

Place the zucchini halves on a baking dish. Fill the zucchini boats with the Mediterranean turkey mixture.

Bake in a preheated oven for 20-25 minutes, or until the zucchini softens.

Garnish with fresh parsley and serve with lemon wedges as preferred.

Benefits for Menopausal Women:

1. Lean Protein Source: Lean ground turkey or chicken provides a protein source

essential for muscle health during menopause.

2. Omega-3 Fatty Acids: If using turkey, choose ground turkey with omega-3 fatty acids for additional anti-inflammatory benefits.

3. Healthy Fats: Kalamata olives and olive oil contribute monounsaturated fats, supporting heart health and providing a satisfying element to the dish.

4. Bone Health: Feta cheese adds a touch of calcium, vital

for maintaining bone health during menopause.

5. Antioxidant-rich: Cherry tomatoes and olives are rich in antioxidants, helping combat oxidative stress associated with hormonal changes.

6. Herbs for Flavor and Health: Dried oregano and basil not only enhance flavor but also offer potential anti-inflammatory and digestive benefits.

7. Low-Carb Option: Zucchini boats provide a low-carb alternative, suitable for women

focusing on managing carbohydrate intake during menopause.

8. Colorful Nutrient Mix: The variety of colorful vegetables provides a mix of vitamins, minerals, and phytonutrients, supporting overall well-being.

9. Hydration Support: Zucchini has high water content, contributing to hydration, which is essential for overall health and can be particularly beneficial during menopause.

The Mediterranean Zucchini Boats offers a simple yet delicious way to incorporate a variety of nutrients into a meal, making it a practical and enjoyable option for women in the menopausal phase.

Incorporating these Mediterranean Zucchini Boats into a menopausal woman's diet not only provides a burst of flavor but also addresses specific nutritional needs, making it a delightful and health-conscious choice during this transformative stage of life.

9. Turmeric-Ginger Tea:

Ingredients:

1 tablespoon honey or maple syrup (optional sweetness)

1 tablespoon lemon juice (optional)

2 cups water

Pinch of black pepper (improves turmeric absorption)

Fresh mint leaves for garnish (optional)

Preparation:

In a small saucepan, bring 2 cups of water to a simmer.

Add ground turmeric or grated fresh turmeric and grated ginger to the simmering water.

Allow the mixture to simmer for about 7-10 minutes, ensuring the flavors are infused into the water.

If using, add honey or maple syrup for sweetness and lemon juice for a

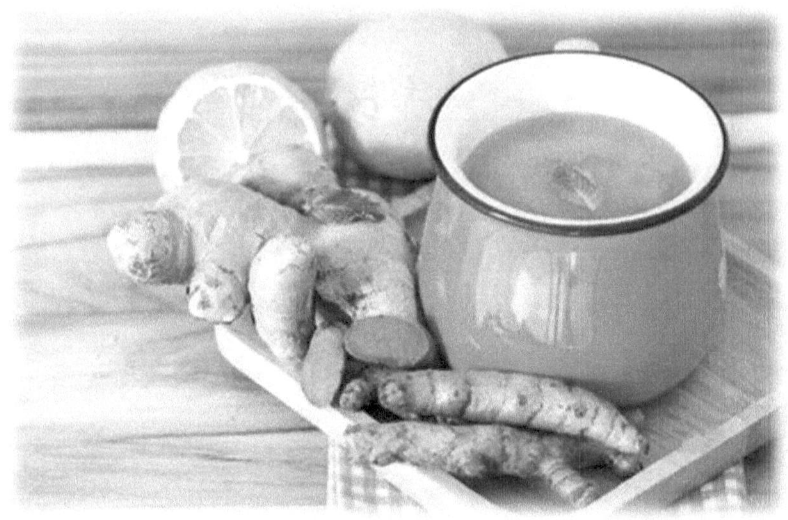

citrusy twist. Stir until well combined.

Remove the saucepan from heat and strain the tea to remove the turmeric and ginger particles.

Pour the tea into your favorite mug and garnish with fresh mint leaves if desired.

Benefits for Menopausal Women:

1. Anti-Inflammatory Properties: Turmeric includes curcumin, which is believed to reduce inflammation. This can help manage inflammation related with menopausal symptoms.

2. Digestive Health: Ginger aids in digestion and can alleviate digestive discomfort, which may become more prevalent during menopause.

3. Immune Support: The combination of turmeric and ginger provides immune-boosting properties, supporting

overall health during this phase.

4. Natural Antioxidants: Turmeric and ginger are rich in antioxidants, helping combat oxidative stress linked to hormonal changes.

5. Warmth and Comfort: A warm beverage like turmeric-ginger tea provides comfort and relaxation, potentially easing stress and promoting emotional well-being.

6. Hydration: Staying well-hydrated is crucial during menopause, and turmeric-ginger tea offers a flavorful option without added caffeine.

7. Joint and Muscle Support: Turmeric is believed to have benefits for joint health, which can be particularly relevant as women age and experience changes in joint function.
8. Menopausal Symptom Management: Some women find relief from symptoms like hot flashes and mood swings through the anti-inflammatory and soothing properties of turmeric-ginger tea.

Turmeric-ginger tea is a comforting and healthful addition to a menopausal woman's routine, offering a range of potential benefits for both physical and emotional well-being.

10. Berry-Almond Overnight Oats:

Ingredients:

1 tablespoon honey or maple syrup (optional sweetness)

1/2 cup rolled oats

1/2 cup unsweetened almond milk

1/4 cup Greek yogurt

1/2 cup mixed berries (strawberries, blueberries, raspberries)

1 tablespoon almond butter

1 teaspoon chia seeds

Sliced almonds for topping

Fresh mint leaves for garnish (optional)

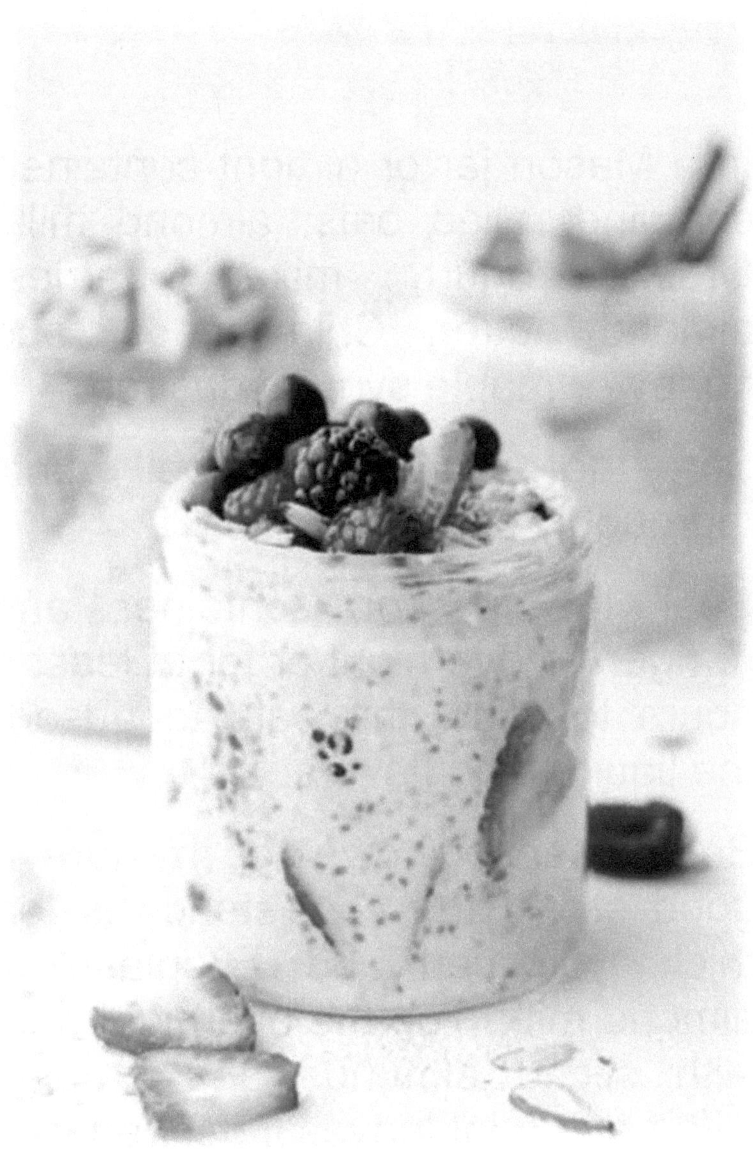

Preparation:

In a Mason jar or airtight container, combine rolled oats, almond milk, Greek yogurt, mixed berries, almond butter, Chia seeds, and honey or maple syrup if desired.

Stir the ingredients well until thoroughly combined.

Seal the jar or container and refrigerate overnight or for at least 4 hours to allow the oats to absorb the liquids and flavors.

Before serving, give the mixture a good stir. If the consistency is too thick, you can add a splash of almond milk. Top the overnight oats with sliced almonds and garnish with fresh mint leaves if desired.

1. Whole Grains for Sustained Energy: Rolled oats provides complex carbohydrates, offering sustained energy throughout the day, which can be beneficial for managing fatigue during menopause.

2. Plant-Based Protein: Greek yogurt and almond butter contribute plant-based protein, essential for muscle health and overall well-being.

3. Healthy Fats: Almond butter and sliced almonds provide healthy fats, supporting heart

health and adding a satisfying element to the meal.

4. Antioxidant-Rich Berries: Mixed berries are rich in antioxidants, combating oxidative stress and supporting overall health during menopause.

5. Omega-3 Fatty Acids: Chia seeds add omega-3 fatty acids, which may have anti-inflammatory benefits and support brain health.

6. Digestive Health: The combination of fiber from oats and chia seeds supports digestive health, potentially

alleviating digestive discomfort associated with hormonal changes.

7. Calcium for Bone Health: Greek yogurt contributes calcium, essential for maintaining bone health during menopause.

8. Natural Sweetness: Honey or maple syrup adds natural sweetness without the need for excessive added sugars, helping manage sugar intake.

9. Convenience and Time-Saving: Overnight oats are a convenient and time-saving

breakfast option, allowing women to prioritize

10. Customizable: This recipe is easily customizable with various toppings or additional ingredients based on individual preferences and dietary needs.

Berry-Almond Overnight Oats offer a delicious and nutrient-dense breakfast option tailored to the specific health considerations of women navigating the menopausal transition

11. Pesto Chicken with Roasted Vegetables:

Ingredients:

2 boneless, skinless chicken breasts

1/4 cup pesto sauce (store-bought or homemade)

1 red bell pepper, sliced

1 yellow bell pepper, sliced

1 Courgette or Zucchini, sliced

2 tablespoons olive oil

Fresh basil for garnish (optional)

1 cup cherry tomatoes.

Preparation:

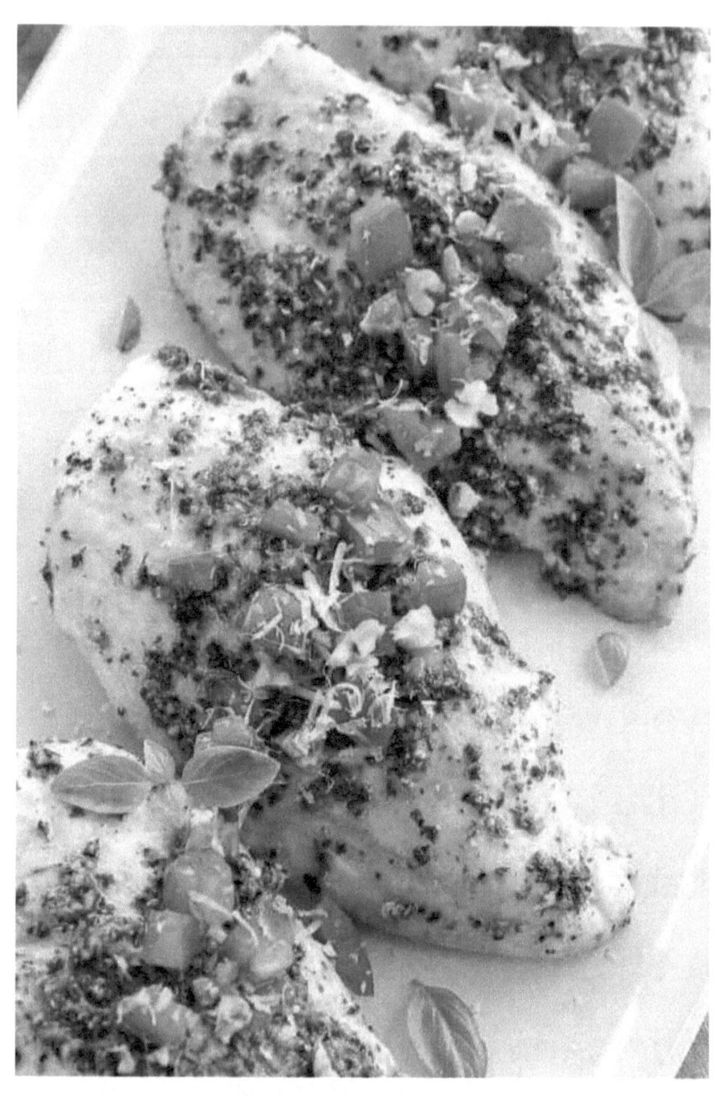

Preheat the oven to 400°F (200°C).

Place the chicken breasts on a baking sheet lined with parchment paper.

Spread pesto sauce evenly over each chicken breast.

In a bowl, toss the sliced bell peppers, zucchini, and cherry tomatoes with olive oil, salt, and pepper.

Place the seasoned veggies around the chicken on the baking sheet.

Roast in the preheated oven for 20-25 minutes, or until the chicken is fully cooked and the vegetables are soft, flipping occasionally to ensure uniform cooking.

Garnish with fresh basil before serving.

Benefits for Menopausal Women:

1. Lean Protein Source: Chicken breasts offer a lean protein source crucial for maintaining muscle health during menopause.

2. Healthy Fats: Pesto sauce, made with ingredients like basil, pine nuts, and olive oil, provides heart-healthy monounsaturated fats.

3. Colorful Vegetables for Nutrients: Bell peppers, zucchini, and cherry tomatoes are rich in vitamins, minerals, and antioxidants, supporting overall well-being.

4. Anti-Inflammatory Properties: Basil in the pesto sauce contains compounds with potential anti-inflammatory benefits, aiding in managing inflammation associated with menopausal symptoms.

5. Digestive Health: The fiber from vegetables contributes to digestive health, potentially alleviating digestive discomfort.

6. Versatile and Time-Efficient: This one-pan dish is versatile and time-efficient, making it a convenient option for busy schedules during menopause.

7. Low-Carb Option: The focus on vegetables and lean protein makes this dish a lower-carb option, suitable for those managing carbohydrate intake.

8. Customizable: Feel free to adjust the types of vegetables or experiment with different homemade pesto variations to suit personal preferences.

Pesto Chicken with Roasted Vegetables is a flavorful and nutritious dish designed to provide essential nutrients while addressing specific health considerations for women during the menopausal transition.

12. Spinach and Feta Stuffed Mushrooms:

Ingredients:

12 large mushrooms, cleaned and stems removed

1 cup fresh spinach, chopped

1/2 cup feta cheese, crumbled

2 cloves garlic, minced

1 tablespoon olive oil

Salt and pepper to taste

Fresh parsley for garnish (optional)

Preparation:

Preheat the oven to 375°F (190°C).

In a pan, heat olive oil over medium heat. Add the minced garlic and cook until fragrant.

Cook the chopped spinach until it has wilted.

Remove the skillet from the heat and mix in the crumbled feta cheese.

Season with salt and pepper to taste.

Arrange the filled mushrooms on a baking sheet lined with parchment paper.

Bake in a preheated oven for 15-20 minutes, or until the mushrooms are soft and the filling is golden brown.

Bake in the preheated oven for 15-20 minutes or until the mushrooms

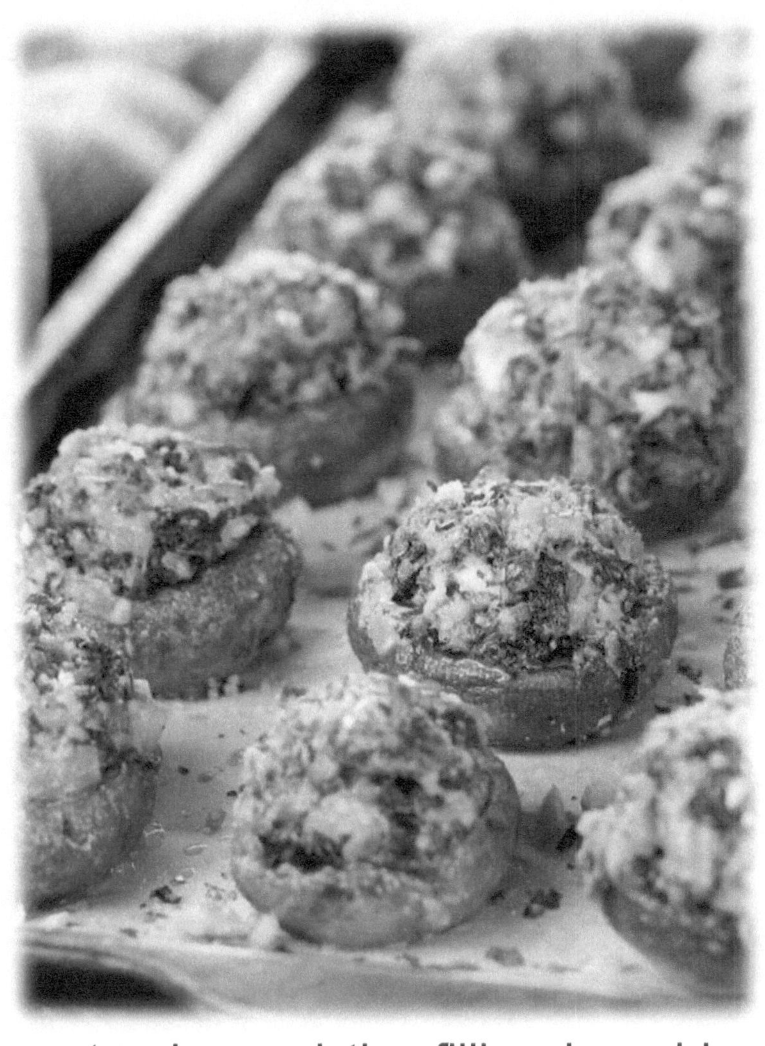

are tender and the filling is golden brown.

87

Garnish with fresh parsley if desired before serving.

Benefits to Menopausal Women:

1. Calcium for Bone Health: Feta cheese is a source of calcium, which is crucial for maintaining bone health during menopause.

2. Iron-Rich Spinach: Spinach provides iron, helping combat the risk of anemia that can occur during menopause.

3. Protein and Fiber: Both feta cheese and spinach contribute

protein and fiber, promoting satiety and supporting digestive health.

4. Low-Calorie Option: Stuffed mushrooms offer a flavorful and low-calorie option, suitable for women managing their weight during menopause.

5. Antioxidants: Spinach is rich in antioxidants that may help combat oxidative stress associated with hormonal changes.

6. Versatile and Customizable: This recipe is versatile, allowing for variations in herbs

or additional ingredients according to personal taste.

7. Easy to Prepare: Stuffed mushrooms are easy to prepare and can be served as an appetizer or a light meal, catering to women with varied dietary preferences.

Spinach and Feta Stuffed Mushrooms provide a delicious and nutrient-dense option that aligns with the nutritional needs of women

13. Coconut-Lime Shrimp Skewers:

Ingredients:

1 pound large shrimp, peeled and deveined

1/2 cup coconut milk

Zest and juice of 1 lime

2 tablespoons coconut oil, melted

2 cloves garlic, minced

1 teaspoon chili flakes

1 tablespoon freshly chopped cilantro (optional for garnish)

Salt and pepper to taste

Wooden or metal skewers

91

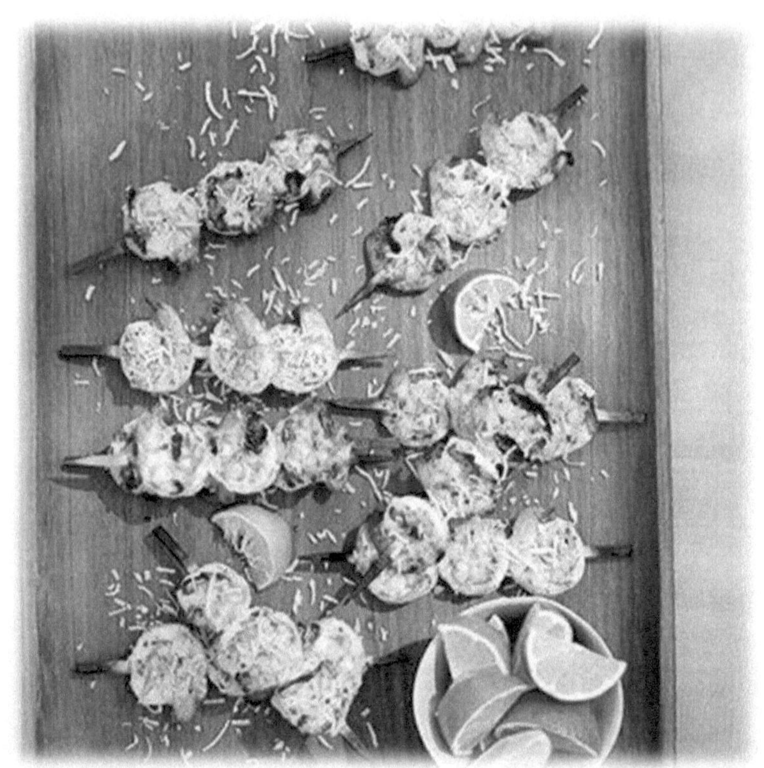

To prevent burning, soak the wooden skewers in water for at least 30 minutes.

In a bowl, combine coconut milk, lime zest, lime juice, melted

92

coconut oil, minced garlic, chili flakes, salt, and pepper.

Add the peeled and deveined shrimp to the marinade, ensuring they are well-coated. Let it marinate for at least 30 minutes in the refrigerator.

Preheat the grill or grill pan over medium-high heat.

Thread the marinated shrimp onto skewers.

Grill the shrimp skewers for 2-3 minutes per side or until they are opaque and cooked through.

Garnish with freshly chopped cilantro before serving.

Benefits for Menopausal Women:

1. Omega-3 Fatty Acids: Shrimp is a source of omega-3 fatty acids, supporting heart health and potentially alleviating menopausal symptoms.

2. Lean Protein: Shrimp provides lean protein essential for muscle health and overall well-being during menopause.

3. Coconut Milk for Healthy Fats: Coconut milk contributes healthy fats, offering a satiating and flavorful element to the dish.

4. Vitamin C from Lime: Lime provides vitamin C, supporting

the immune system and promoting overall health.

5. Low in Calories: Shrimp is relatively low in calories, making it a suitable option for women managing their weight during menopause.

6. Quick and Easy Preparation: This recipe is quick and easy to prepare, making it a convenient choice for busy schedules.

7. Customizable Heat Level: Adjust the amount of chili flakes to suit personal taste preferences for spiciness.

Coconut-lime shrimp skewers offer a delightful blend of flavors and nutrients, making them a tasty and health-conscious option for women navigating the menopausal transition.

14. Almond Butter and Banana Smoothie Bowl:

Ingredients:

2 frozen bananas, sliced

1/4 cup almond butter

1 cup almond milk (unsweetened)

1 tablespoon chia seeds

1 tablespoon of honey or maple syrup (optional for sweetness)

Toppings: Sliced bananas, almonds, granola, and a drizzle of almond butter

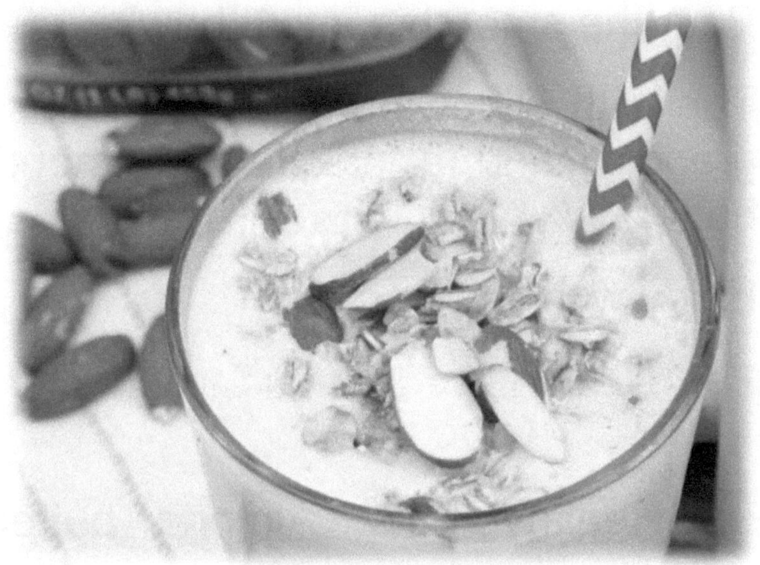

Preparation:

In a blender, combine frozen banana slices, almond butter, almond milk, chia seeds, and honey or maple syrup.

97

Blend until smooth and creamy, adding more almond milk if needed to reach the desired consistency.

Pour the smoothie into a bowl.

Top with sliced bananas, almonds, granola, and a drizzle of almond butter.

Enjoy with a spoon!

Benefits for Menopausal Women:

1. Healthy Fats: Almond butter provides healthy monounsaturated fats, supporting heart health and satiety.

2. Potassium from Bananas: Bananas are a good source of

potassium, which is essential for maintaining electrolyte balance and supporting cardiovascular health.

3. Plant-Based Protein: Almond butter and chia seeds contribute plant-based protein, aiding in muscle health during menopause.

4. Fiber-rich Chia Seeds: Chia seeds are rich in fiber, promoting digestive health and helping manage blood sugar levels.

5. Calcium and Vitamin D from Almond Milk: Almond milk

fortified with calcium and vitamin D contributes to bone health during menopause.

6. Energy-Boosting Carbohydrates: Bananas provide natural sugars and carbohydrates for a quick energy boost.

7. Customizable Toppings: The variety of toppings allows for customization based on taste preferences and nutritional needs.

8. Soothing and Refreshing: A smoothie bowl is a soothing and refreshing option,

especially for women experiencing hot flashes during menopause.

Almond Butter and Banana Smoothie Bowl is a nutrient-dense and delicious option that aligns with the specific nutritional needs of women navigating the menopausal transition.

15. Eggplant and Chickpea Curry:

Ingredients:

1large eggplant, diced
1 can chickpeas, drained / rinsed

1 onion, finely chopped

2 cloves garlic, minced

1 tablespoon ginger, grated

1 can diced tomatoes

1 can coconut milk

2 tablespoons curry powder

1 teaspoon turmeric

1 teaspoon cumin

1 teaspoon coriander

1/2 tsp red pepper flakes (to taste)

Salt and pepper to taste

Fresh cilantro for garnish

Cooked brown rice or quinoa for serving

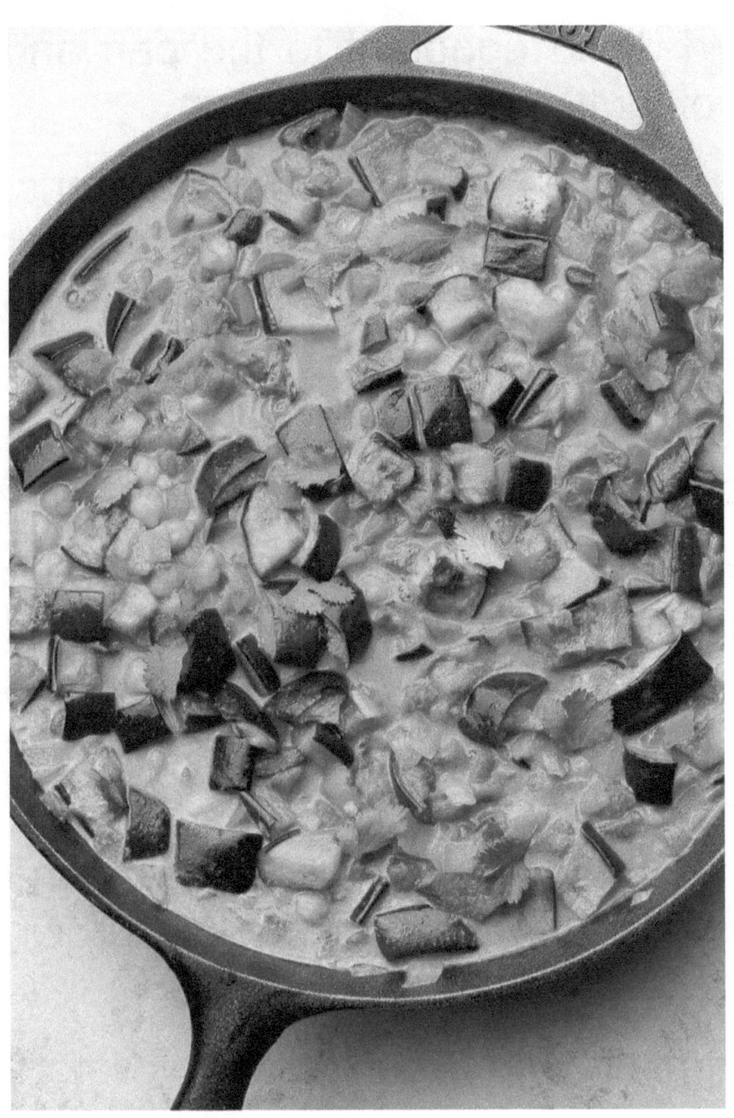

In a large pan, sauté

103

Add diced eggplant to the pan and cook until it begins to brown.

Stir in the curry powder, turmeric, cumin, coriander, and red pepper flakes, coating the vegetables evenly.

Pour in the diced tomatoes and coconut milk, stirring well.

Add the drained chickpeas to the mixture and season with salt and pepper. Simmer for 15-20 minutes until the eggplant is tender and the flavors meld.

Adjust seasoning to taste, and serve the curry over cooked brown rice or quinoa.

Garnish with fresh cilantro before serving.

Benefits for Menopausal Women:

1. Plant-Based Protein: Chickpeas provide plant-based protein, essential for muscle health and overall well-being during menopause.

2. Fiber-rich Eggplant: Eggplant is rich in fiber, supporting digestive health and promoting satiety.

3. Anti-Inflammatory Spices: Turmeric, cumin, and coriander have anti-inflammatory properties that may help alleviate symptoms associated with menopause.

4. Healthy Fats from Coconut Milk: Coconut milk contributes healthy fats, providing a satisfying and flavorful element to the dish.

5. Balanced Macronutrients: The combination of protein, fiber, and healthy fats creates a well-balanced meal suitable for women managing their weight during menopause.

6. Bone Health Support: Calcium and phosphorus from chickpeas contribute to bone health.

7. Customizable Spice Level: The red pepper flakes can be adjusted according to personal preference for spiciness.

8. Vegetarian Option: This vegetarian curry offers a plant-based alternative for women seeking meatless meals during menopause.

Eggplant and chickpea curry is a nourishing and flavorful dish designed to provide essential nutrients while addressing specific health considerations for women during the menopausal transition.

16. Chia Seed Pudding with Berries:

Ingredients:

1/4 cup chia seeds

1 cup almond milk (unsweetened)

1 tablespoon maple syrup or honey

1/2 teaspoon vanilla extract

Mixed berries (strawberries, blueberries, raspberries) for topping

Sliced almonds for garnish (optional)

Mint leaves for garnish (optional)

Preparation:

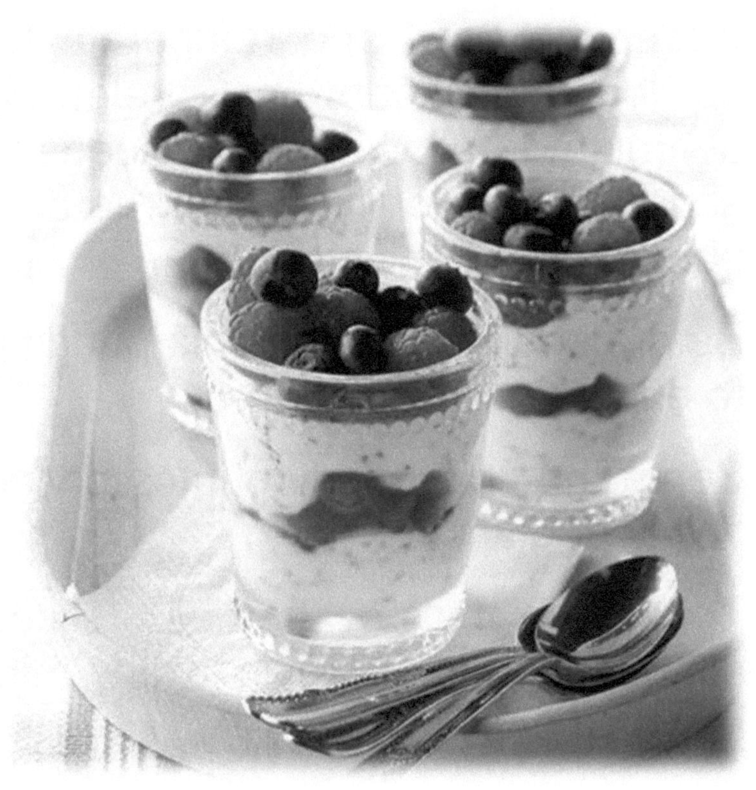

In a bowl, combine chia seeds, almond milk, maple syrup or honey, and vanilla extract.

Whisk the ingredients together, ensuring the chia seeds are well dispersed in the mixture.

Cover the bowl and refrigerate for at least 4 hours or preferably overnight to allow the chia seeds to absorb the liquid and create a pudding-like consistency.

Before serving, stir the chia pudding to ensure an even texture.

Serve the chia pudding into serving bowls or glasses.

Top with mixed berries, sliced almonds, and garnish with mint leaves if desired.

Benefits to Menopausal Women:

1. Omega-3 Fatty Acids: Chia seeds are rich in omega-3 fatty acids, which may help support

heart health and manage inflammation during menopause.

2. Fiber-Rich Pudding: Chia seeds are an excellent source of soluble fiber, promoting digestive health and helping manage cholesterol levels.

3. Plant-Based Protein: Chia seeds provide plant-based protein, supporting muscle health and overall well-being.

4. Low-Glycemic Sweetener: Maple syrup or honey adds sweetness without causing a rapid spike in blood sugar

levels, making it suitable for women managing their blood sugar during menopause.

5. Antioxidant-Rich Berries: Mixed berries are rich in antioxidants, which play a role in combating oxidative stress associated with hormonal changes.

6. Bone Health Support: Almond milk may be fortified with calcium and vitamin D, contributing to bone health during menopause.

7. Satisfying and Nutrient-Dense: Chia seed pudding is a satisfying and nutrient-dense

option, offering a balance of healthy fats, protein, and carbohydrates.

Chia Seed Pudding with Berries is a delightful and nutritious treat designed to provide essential nutrients while addressing specific health considerations for women during the menopausal transition.

17. Baked Cod with Lemon-Herb Crust:

Ingredients:

4 cod fillets

1/2 cup breadcrumbs (whole-grain for added fiber)

Zest of 1 lemon

2 tablespoons fresh parsley, finely chopped

1 tablespoon fresh dill, finely chopped

2 tablespoons olive oil

1 clove garlic, minced

Salt and pepper to taste

Lemon wedges for serving

Preparation:

Preheat the oven to 400°F (200°C).

In a bowl, combine breadcrumbs, lemon zest, chopped parsley, chopped dill, minced garlic, olive oil, salt, and pepper. To make the herb crust, combine all the ingredients thoroughly.

Place the cod fillets on a baking sheet lined with parchment paper. Press the herb crust mixture onto the top of each cod fillet, ensuring an even coating.

Bake in a pre-heated oven for 12–15 minutes, or until the cod is cooked through, and the crust is golden brown.

Serve the baked cod with lemon wedges on the side.

Benefits for Menopausal Women:

Omega-3 Fatty Acids: Cod is a lean fish that provides omega-3 fatty acids, supporting heart health and potentially alleviating menopausal symptoms.

1. Lean Protein: Cod is a good source of lean protein, essential for muscle health and overall well-being.

2. Whole-Grain Fiber: Using whole-grain breadcrumbs adds fiber to the dish, supporting digestive health and satiety.

3. Herbs for Flavor and Antioxidants: Fresh parsley and dill not only enhance flavor but also provide antioxidants that may combat oxidative stress.

4. Heart-Healthy Olive Oil: Olive oil in the herb crust contributes

heart-healthy monounsaturated fats.

5. Low-Calorie Option: Baked cod is a low-calorie option, suitable for women managing their weight during menopause.

6. Quick and Easy Preparation: This recipe is quick and easy to prepare, making it a convenient choice for busy schedules.

Baked Cod with Lemon-Herb Crust offers a delicious and health-conscious option, incorporating key nutrients that align with the specific health needs of women during the menopausal transition.

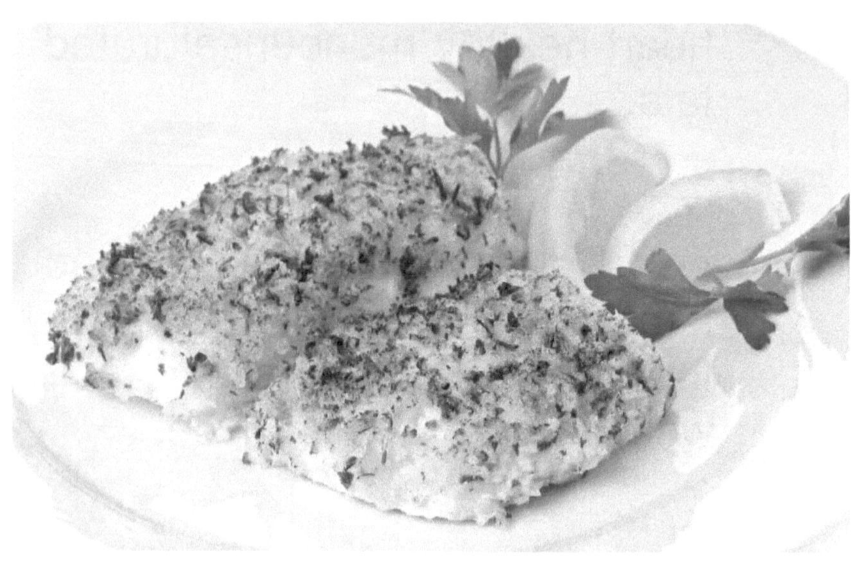

18. Greek Yogurt Parfait with Nuts and Berries:

Ingredients:

1 cup Greek yogurt (unsweetened)

Mixed berries (strawberries, blueberries, raspberries)

1/4 cup mixed nuts (almonds, walnuts, or pistachios), chopped

Honey or maple syrup for drizzling

Granola (optional for added crunch)

Preparation:

In a glass or dish, place Greek yogurt at the bottom.

Put a layer of mixed berries on top of the yogurt.

Sprinkle some chopped mixed nuts over the fruit.

Repeat the layers until the glass or bowl is full.

Drizzle honey or maple syrup over the top.

Optionally, sprinkle granola for added texture and flavor.

Serve immediately, and enjoy!

Benefits for Menopausal Women:

1. Protein-Packed Greek Yogurt: Greek yogurt is rich in protein, supporting muscle health during menopause.

2. Antioxidant-rich Berries: Mixed berries provide antioxidants that may help combat oxidative stress associated with hormonal changes.

3. Healthy Fats from Nuts: Mixed nuts contribute healthy fats, providing satiety and supporting overall well-being.

4. Bone Health Support: Greek yogurt may contain calcium and vitamin D, important for maintaining bone health during menopause.

5. Low-Glycemic Sweetener: Drizzling honey or maple syrup adds sweetness without causing a rapid spike in blood sugar levels.

6. Versatile and Customizable: This parfait is versatile, allowing for variations based on personal taste preferences and nutritional needs.

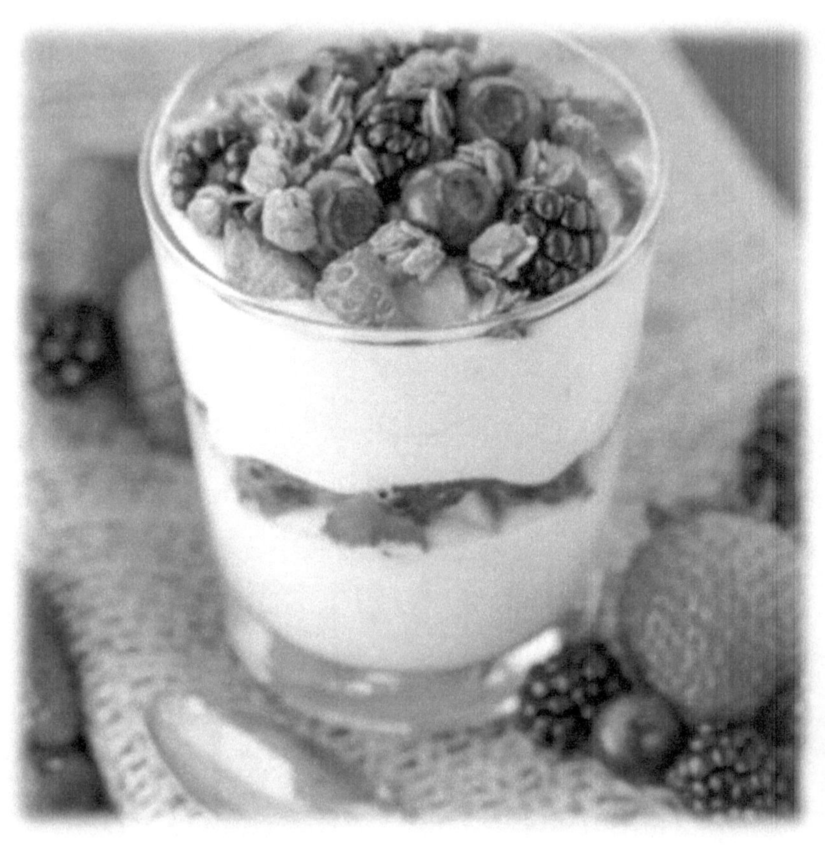

19. Lentil and Vegetable Soup:

Ingredients:

1 cup dried lentils, rinsed

1 onion, diced

2 carrots, sliced

2 celery stalks, chopped

3 cloves garlic, minced

1 can diced tomatoes

6 cups vegetable broth

1 teaspoon ground cumin

1 teaspoon smoked paprika

1/2 teaspoon turmeric

Salt and pepper to taste

Fresh parsley for garnish

Preparation:

In a large pot, sauté the diced onion, carrots, celery, and minced garlic until softened.

Add dried lentils, diced tomatoes, vegetable broth, cumin, smoked paprika, turmeric, salt, and pepper. Bring to a boil.

Reduce the heat and boil for 25–30 minutes, or until the lentils are cooked.

Adjust seasoning to taste and garnish with fresh parsley before serving.

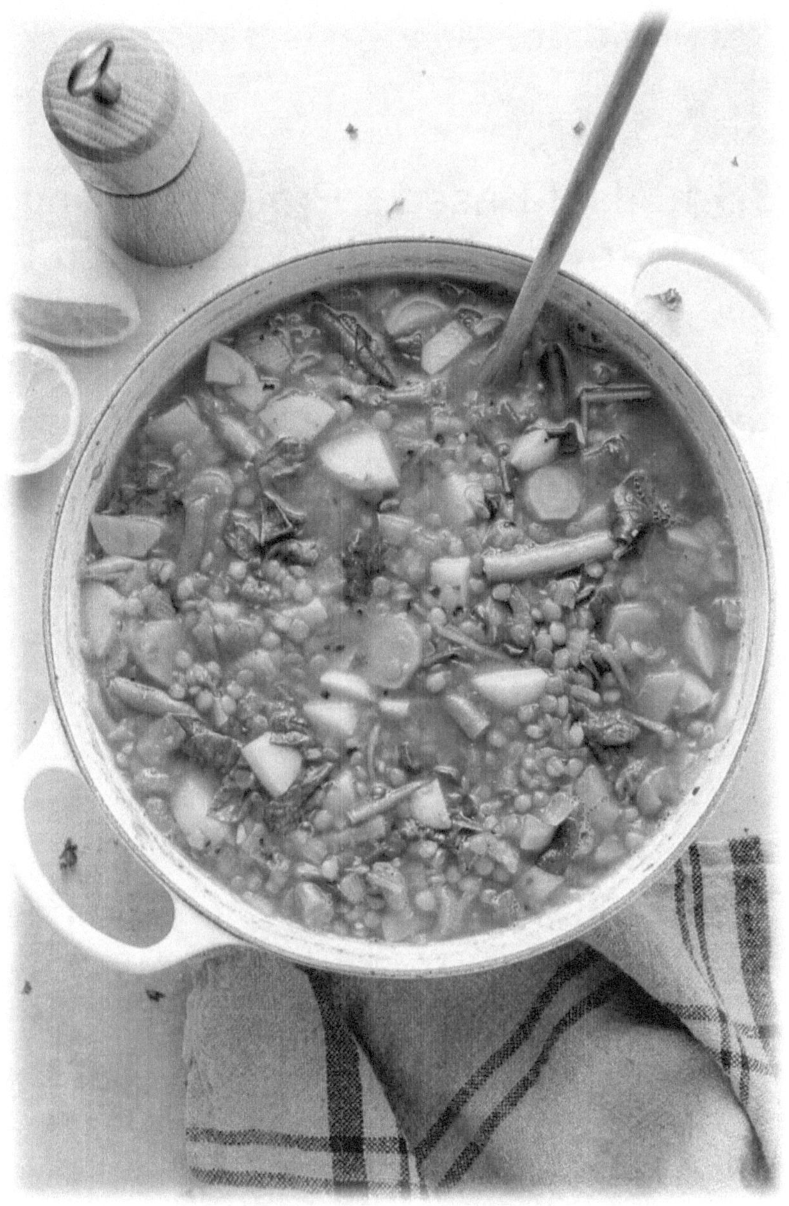

1. Plant-Based Protein: Lentils provide plant-based protein, essential for muscle health and overall well-being during menopause.

2. Fiber-Rich Soup: Lentils and vegetables contribute fiber, promoting digestive health and satiety.

3. Anti-Inflammatory Spices: Cumin, smoked paprika, and turmeric have anti-inflammatory properties that may help alleviate symptoms associated with menopause.

4. Low-Calorie Option: Lentil and vegetable soup is a nutrient-dense and low-calorie option suitable for women managing their weight during menopause.

5. Versatile and Filling: This soup is versatile and can be customized with additional vegetables or herbs based on personal preference.

20. Roasted Brussels sprouts with Balsamic Glaze:

Ingredients:

127

1 pound Brussels sprouts, trimmed and halved

2 tablespoons olive oil

Salt and pepper to taste

2 tablespoons balsamic glaze

Preparation:

Preheat the oven to 400°F (200°C).

In a bowl, combine Brussels sprouts, olive oil, salt, and pepper.

Place the Brussels sprouts on a baking sheet in a single layer.

Roast in a preheated oven for 20–25 minutes, or until crispy and golden brown.

Drizzle balsamic glaze over the roasted Brussels sprouts before serving

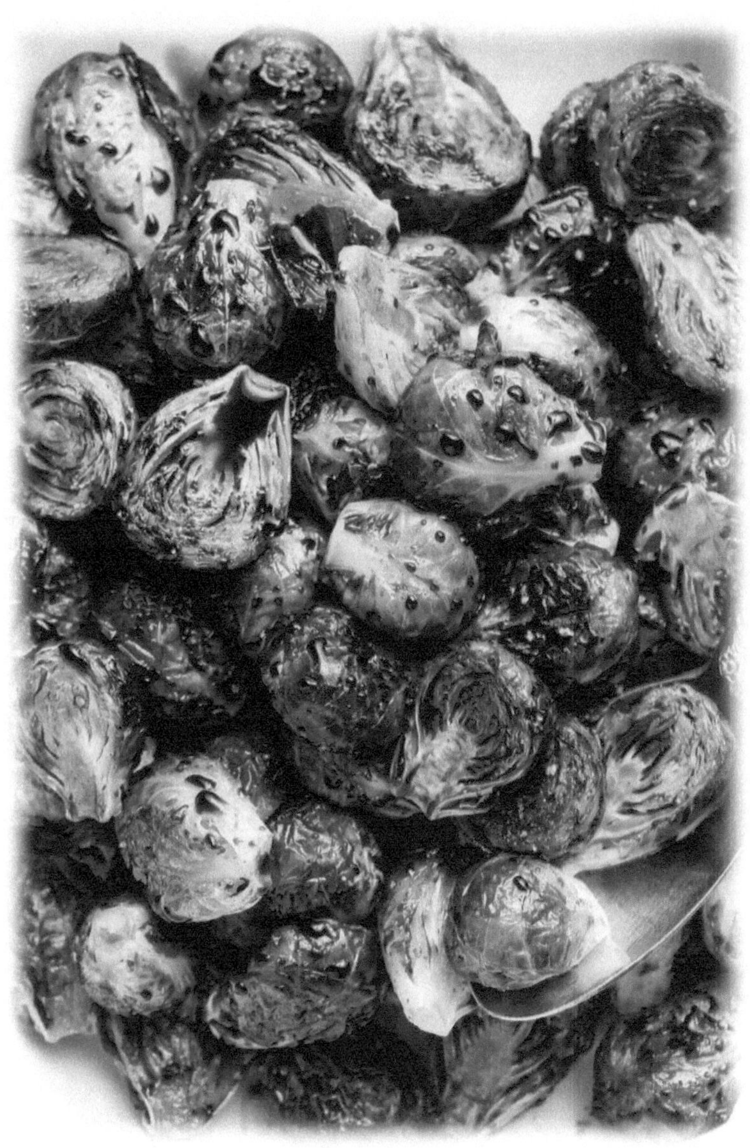

1. Fiber-Rich Brussels Sprouts: Brussels sprouts provide fiber, supporting digestive health and promoting satiety.

2. Vitamin C: Brussels sprouts are rich in vitamin C, which supports the immune system and overall health.

3. Heart-Healthy Olive Oil: Olive oil used in roasting contributes heart-healthy monounsaturated fats.

4. Low-Calorie and Nutrient-Dense: Roasted Brussels sprouts are a low-calorie option

packed with essential nutrients, suitable for women managing their weight during menopause.

5. Quick and Easy Side Dish: This recipe is quick and easy to prepare, making it a convenient and nutritious side dish.

Conclusion

In the culinary journey through menopause, "Nourish & Thrive" emerges not just as a compilation of delicious dishes but also as a comprehensive guide to navigating this transforming time. Beyond the kitchen, the book dives into lifestyle choices and nutritional advice, serving as a full reference for women going through menopause.

As we embark on the culinary and wellness adventure together, "Nourish & Thrive" aims to be more than a cookbook; it aspires to be a trusted companion, equipping you not only with tools for the kitchen but also with the knowledge to make informed choices that positively impact your menopausal transition.

This book celebrates energy, balance, and the robust woman emerging from the experience of menopause. This cookbook contains delicious and simple recipes as well as a wealth of wellness information.

As you read through the culinary pleasures and wellness lessons included in these pages, may "Nourish & Thrive" serve as a source of empowerment for you, allowing you to tackle this challenge with bravery and embrace the vibrant lady you will become. Here's to feeding your body, mind, and spirit as you navigate menopause, complete with tasty recipes, holistic lifestyle options, delicious and simple foods to select from, and an abundance of health information. As you close the cover, let it symbolize not just the end of a book but the beginning of a newfound connection with your own well-being. This book is more than a guide; it's a testament to your journey, marked by flavorful dishes, mindful choices, and the unwavering spirit that defines the remarkable woman navigating through menopause.

The end of "Nourish & Thrive" is not a farewell; rather, it is an invitation to bring the knowledge learned, recipes treasured, and empowerment encouraged into the chapters of your own life.

Embrace the vibrancy within you, savor the flavors of a well-nourished life, and continue thriving through the transformative and empowering experience of menopause. Cheers to a life filled with vitality, balance, and the endless possibilities that await you beyond these pages.

Happy Cooking!!!